walk

The path to a more mindful life

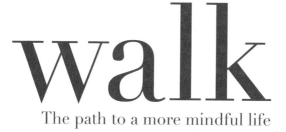

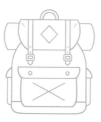

sholto radford

Illustrations by Robbie Porter

quadrille

'In every walk
with Nature one
receives far more
than he seeks.'

JOHN MUIR

CONTENTS

INTRODUCTION

I believe there is a quiet voice within all of us, a voice that speaks to the mystery of this life, that whispers of a simplicity and the possibility of a connection to the fundamental raw aliveness in our nature; a voice that questions our efforts to order and better our lives, to work through the never-ending tasks on our to-do lists and face the baffling array of choices, enticements and distractions of life, where the world is seemingly at our fingertips. This voice may be loud and clear, or it may be buried deep down, only surfacing occasionally, raising itself above the cacophony of all of the things we have to get done today.

How do we answer? We could simply put on our shoes and leave everything behind us – step outside and walk. Yet to escape but rather to return – to reconnect with something more fundamental to who we are than our inbox. Walking has the potential to nourish us physically and emotionally, to inspire us with ideas, creativity and insights. It can help us feel more connected to the natural world, give us a sense of perspective, meaning, wonder or presence. And when we step back through the door, perhaps we will have more clarity and inspiration as we meet both the undeniable challenges and the joys of life.

WALKING LEADS US INTO AN ENCOUNTER WITH THE WORLD

Whether we are exploring new places or walking on familiar turf, we pass other people, trees and plants, animals and human creations. We are exposed to the elements through the changing weather and seasons, and the natural rhythms of day and night. It may take us to dramatic places, mountains, rivers, forests, beaches and cities. It is not possible to separate the act of walking from what we see, hear, feel, touch and are touched by. Walking is a conversation with the world and ourselves within it.

This book explores this territory with the understanding that walking can also be more than just a physical activity, a way of getting from A to B or experiencing an unfamiliar place. It can become an art or practice, a conscious way of exploring our human experience, opening to our lives and cultivating the capacity of mindful awareness and well-being.

It is my hope that this book will engage this voice within us, and perhaps spark some curiosity about the potential of this seemingly simple act of movement. Ultimately, I hope it inspires you to get out there and walk.

APPROACHING THIS BOOK

Our bodies evolved to move. The act of walking benefits our physical health and well-being and it can be a great way of looking after our bodies and minds.

Beyond this, this book offers exercises and practices to support readers in walking as a conscious practice. Walking becomes a way to cultivate awareness, to open ourselves more fully to our senses and the world around us, to reflect on our connection to the natural world and find space to settle into a more present, focussed, mindful way of being.

No amount of reading can do this for us. To experience the benefits requires you to get out there and explore this for yourself. I hope this book provides inspiration and encouragement, but ultimately it is up to you. The capacity to be more present can take practice and can be a subtle process; I encourage you to approach the practices with curiosity and patience. If we try too hard or have fixed expectations, goals and judgements, then paradoxically we may simply be stepping back into the mode of 'doing', of striving for something other than what is here: the antithesis of mindfulness.

A helpful way to approach the practices is as if there is no end goal, nothing to be reached, achieved or improved upon. In this way, as we walk, we are open to what is really happening for us moment by moment rather than limited by our thoughts of what our experience should be.

The ideas and practices in this book are just suggestions, so only take on or do what feels right for you. At the same time I encourage you to be curious and open-minded. It seems that in order to see things in a fresh light we often have to let go of our conditioned views, of what we think we already know, and only by doing this is there the potential for new learning to arise.

A disability or injury may mean that walking is difficult for you or not even possible. If so, I encourage you to be creative and to explore what is possible. I believe that much of this book will still be relevant. It may require more consideration of where you choose to go, and some adaptations to the practices, but the essence of getting out into the world, being open and curious to what is around and within us and cultivating awareness is not dependent on your style of movement.

Everyone will have their own physical abilities and limitations, pains, injuries and relationship to walking. It is not the purpose of this book to encourage you to push yourself to new physical limits, but rather to develop awareness, self-care and explore with curiosity what is possible for you without either overdoing it or unnecessarily holding back. If you have specific challenges it may also be wise to seek support from a relevant health professional.

'I only went out for a walk
and finally concluded to
stay out till sundown, for
going out, I found, was
really going in.'

JOHN MUIR

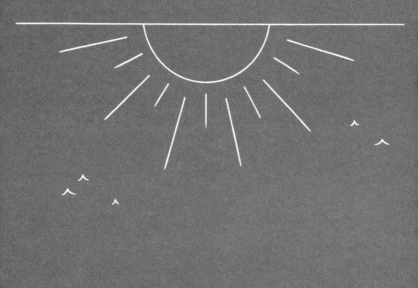

EARLY BEGINNINGS

Our hominid ancestors began the life of bipedalism over six million years ago, and to this day walking on two feet sets humans apart from all other mammals. The reasons for this development are still debated within the scientific community with numerous theories proposed for why we walk in this way. A popular view, the Savanna Theory, argues that changes to the Earth's climate and the associated reduction in forest cover led us to a life on the plains, where walking on two feet allowed us both to move more efficiently than on four legs, and to look out over the long grass for predators and prey. A more recent theory contests this and suggests that bipedalism was present before such dramatic climate change took place and that life on two feet began while early humans were still living in the trees like our orangutan cousins, who have similar knee joints and walk along branches on two feet, using their hands for balance and to collect food.

Despite over six million years of evolution, the back and knee pains common for us humans are still believed to result from our body's incomplete adaptation and its ancestral roots of moving on all fours.

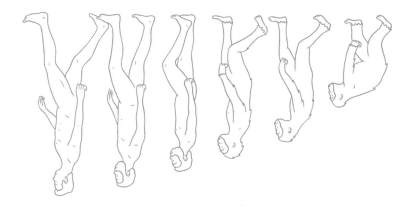

Another significant evolutionary advantage of bipedalism is that it freed our hands. This allowed us to carry food, use tools and weapons and to take on bigger prey. The learning and possibilities available to us through the use of our hands is believed to have played a key role in the development of our brains.

In this sense walking on two feet seems to have been fundamental to the development of human consciousness, the most complex property in our known universe that has given rise to everything mankind has created, and for better or worse has shaped the modern world.

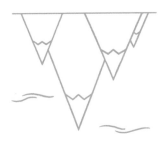

WHY WE WALK

Beyond the evolutionary advantages walking has given us for our survival, it seems to have fulfilled many purposes in human life throughout history. It used to be the only way we could travel, and even in modern Western culture we still use walking as a form of transport. Despite large individual differences, the average healthy person is estimated to take around 7,500 steps in a day – equivalent to five times around the Earth in a lifetime.

The diverse forms and purposes of walking are reflected in our language, with over 60 synonyms for the word 'walk' in English. As well as our primary way of moving around, walking can also be a social activity, a chance to catch up with friends or meet others – to promenade.

People walk to take a break, to get fresh air, for exercise and health, even for sport. It can make us feel more attached to our surroundings and neighbourhoods as well as being an intimate way to explore new places. Some may walk for the challenge, to climb mountains or go on long treks, perhaps partly drawn by an instinctual urge, a throwback to our times of a nomadic lifestyle.

WALKING IS A WAY OF GETTING OUT AND CONNECTING WITH NATURE

It's a way of immersing ourselves in views and experiencing landscapes, rivers, hills, woodlands and beaches. It may be a means to access other passions and interests, such as photography, birdwatching, natural history, geography or geology. Since ancient times people have also walked for spiritual practice or religion: from the pilgrimages of Christianity, Islam, Buddhism and Hinduism, the walkabouts of the Aboriginal Australians, to the rites of passage of the Native Americans. Walking has been highly valued by philosophers, poets and artists as a space for creativity and reflection.

From the Zen monk slowly placing one foot in front of the other in walking meditation to the carefully placed foot of a mountaineer walking on a knife-edge ridge – their own temple – walking crosses cultures, lifestyles and religions. It is a commonality we share as humans.

MOVEMENT AND HEALTH

Our bodies evolved with movement and it is evident that we need to move in order to stay healthy. This was not lost on our ancestors 2,400 years ago, when Hippocrates noted that 'Walking is a man's best medicine'. Through scientific studies we are learning more about the benefits of exercise for our health and well-being. The World Health Organisation recommends that each week we engage with 300 minutes of aerobic activity of moderate intensity, 150 minutes of vigorous activity or a combination of these.

When we think of exercise it is likely that we summon an image of someone clad in sporty clothing, running outside or training in a gym. We overlook walking, which is an effective form of moderately intense activity and can be a valuable way of taking care of ourselves, keeping us healthy in body and mind.

Walking has a number of distinct advantages.

- It is low-impact, so easier on the body than most other forms of exercise and less likely to cause injury.
- It is relatively easy to do whatever your current state of fitness.
- It can easily be built into our days as a way of getting around without requiring us to change clothes or go to a gym.
- It requires nothing more than a good pair of shoes.
- It takes us outside often in natural environments, which has its own advantages (see page 82).

REFLECTIVE PRACTICE

Without needing to judge yourself, reflect on

- What is your relationship to taking care of your body through exercise?
- If you do exercise, what are your motivations and do they seem to support a respect and care for your body whatever its capabilities or limitations?
- If you feel like you would like to exercise more, how might you do this in a healthy way?

RESEARCH SUGGESTS THAT PEOPLE WHO ARE MORE ACTIVE EXPERIENCE THE FOLLOWING:

Higher levels of:

Cardiorespiratory and muscular fitness

Healthy body mass and composition

Weight management

Lower levels of:

Heart disease

Stroke

Type-2 diabetes

Colon and breast cancer

Metabolic syndrome

All-cause mortality

Depression

Arthritis and hip and vertebral fracture

EXERCISE AND THE MIND

There are also psychological benefits to staying active. As we exercise we release endorphins that reduce our perception of pain and lead to positive feelings, improve our mood and help us regulate our stress. When we are physically active we sleep better, which in turn influences our well-being, cognitive function and immune functioning. Exercise also impacts how we feel about ourselves, our sense of self-esteem, body image and accomplishment.

When we walk outside an additional benefit is that exposure to sunlight stimulates the body to produce serotonin, a neurotransmitter that is important in maintaining mood balance.

REFLECTIVE PRACTICE

• What is your relationship to exercising as a way of taking care of how you feel, your mental well-being?

• How do you feel when you exercise. Do you notice any effects such as changes in your mood, energy or sleep?

• When you don't make time for exercise how do you feel?

• What helps to motivate you when your motivation is low?

THE PSYCHOLOGICAL BENEFITS OF EXERCISE:

- Improves mood
- Reduces stress and improves resilience
- Improves self-esteem
- Increases sense of accomplishment and self-satisfaction
- Decreases symptoms of depression
- Increases energy levels
- Improves body image
- Improves memory
- Improves sleep

THE BENEFITS OF NATURE

Perhaps one of the biggest draws of walking to many is that it takes us outside and brings us into contact with the natural world. This contact with nature seems to offer a number of benefits for our health and well-being. Although this may feel intuitive, research has also helped us understand these effects more fully. Even if we are not immersed in wild natural places, having a view of trees or nature from a window or viewing natural scenes can be beneficial.

These findings have led to initiatives to provide community access to natural environments, green up cities and even bring pictures of natural landscapes and plants into work environments and hospitals to promote health and well-being. In Japan, for example, the recognition of the restorative effects of nature has led doctors to prescribe *shinrin-yoku* or forest bathing.

Walking often brings us into contact with the natural world. In a later section of this book there are some ideas and practices for exploring and deepening the connection (see page 84).

BENEFITS OF EXPOSURE TO NATURE:

- Improves mood
- Improves self-esteem
- Reduces anxiety and stress
- Improves psychological well-being
- Increases in cognitive restoration
- Improves perceptions of general health
- Improves physical health
- Increases immunity

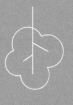

FOREST BATHING

In Japan the practice of *shinrin-yoku* – taking in the forest atmosphere, or 'forest bathing' – first appeared in public health in the 1980s.

The forest bather slowly walks or sits beneath the trees with no aim other than to be open to their senses and breathe in the forest air. The practice is supposed to have calming, rejuvenating effects, improving both physical health and well-being. There is a body of scientific research suggesting that its benefits include boosting immune system function, reducing blood pressure, improving focus, mood and energy levels, reducing blood pressure and stress, and improving sleep. This practice is now beginning to catch on in other countries too.

IS THERE A RIGHT WAY TO WALK?

For most of us walking seems second nature and unless we are experiencing pain or an injury we may not give it a second thought. If this is the case however, you may also be confused by the many and sometimes conflicting approaches to physical movement and posture from experts recommending adjustment through orthopaedic insoles, to those favouring returning to minimal support and barefoot walking. Some recommend focussing on consciously adjusting posture and gait while walking and others suggest that posture and movement are a fundamentally unconscious process and our bodies adjust and respond automatically to injuries to facilitate ease, efficiency and pain free movement. Perhaps there is no one approach for everyone and it may be a matter of seeing what works best for you as an individual.

Through actively paying attention we can begin to notice and identify what is going on in our own body, learn what feels good for us and what seems to cause discomfort or injury. If you have any physical conditions or injuries please consult a specialist.

POSTURE

When you are standing, notice how you are holding your body – are you upright or slouched? Do you notice any tightness or tensing of muscles anywhere in the body? How is your head positioned, is it neutral or tilted to one side, backward or forward? Do you notice any differences between each side of the body, such as in the shoulders, hips or knees? Are your shoulders relaxed and back or tight and held forward? Does the chest feel open or constricted?

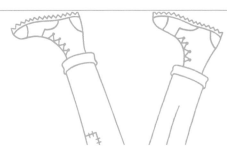

MOVEMENT

When you take a step, which part of the foot contacts the ground first? Do you strike with the heel and then roll the weight towards the ball of your foot, or land with a flat foot?

Is your body weight over the feet as you walk or are you placing the feet further out in front of yourself?

How are you holding your arms when you walk. Do they naturally swing?

Do you notice any areas of pain or tightness as you walk or after exercising?

Becoming intimate with how your body feels as you stand, walk, sit or lie down throughout the day can be a valuable practice in awareness and help connect us with our bodies.

WALKING IN STEEP TERRAIN AND BACKPACKING

Being comfortable walking in steep or rough terrain opens up a world of opportunities to explore rugged, wild and beautiful parts of the world. In order to go out for several days it is usually necessary to carry a backpack, and this can be a further challenge. With time and practice these things become quite natural, but here are some considerations to make this journey easier.

SLOW AND STEADY

On steep ground and long walks, it is helpful to find a pace that you can maintain, rather than getting tired and needing to breath and needing to take a break every ten minutes. Learn to find your rhythm. If it feels too slow at first it is probably right.

PATH OF LEAST RESISTANCE

Learning to read the terrain and choose where you walk is a valuable skill. When the ground gets steep you can find natural zigzags rather than trying to walk straight uphill.

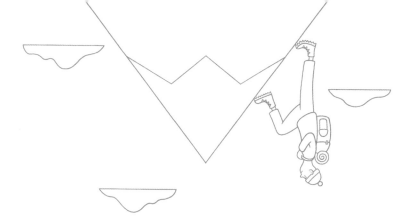

SMALL STEPS

On steep ground it is more efficient and easier on the body to take small steps, keeping the weight under the body, especially when carrying a backpack.

CARRYING A PACK

Some people take the art of saving weight to the extreme but when carrying everything with you for days every gram counts. Walking poles can be especially helpful when carrying packs, as can good boots with ankle support.

CAREFUL FOOT PLACEMENT

In rough ground careful foot placement not only helps with balance and avoids injury but also has the added advantage of helping us to stay present with our experience and the feeling of the body.

WALKING WITH AWARENESS

Present-moment awareness can naturally occur when something like a breathtaking view, a sunset or an encounter with a wild animal captivates our attention and fully engages us. For a moment our concerns drop away and we become acutely present to that moment of experience. Our experience may feel especially vivid, or we may feel joy, contentment or ease.

Besides these incidental moments, present moment awareness – often referred to as mindfulness – is also something that can be intentionally developed or practised. Not only can walking and spending time in the natural world be a place where we can cultivate mindfulness, but in turn mindfulness can be a great companion for walking, allowing us to experience our surroundings more fully and perhaps find more space and nourishment in that time.

'Awareness is like the sun. When it shines on things, they are transformed.'

THICH NHAT HANH

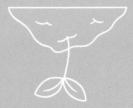

MINDFULNESS AND THE ART OF BEING PRESENT

When our awareness is focussed on our present moment experience in an open and non-judgemental way, this can be described as a state of mindfulness. Naturally our minds spend much of the time focussed on the past or the future, so mindfulness requires a certain level of intention. We need deliberately to bring our awareness to the present moment. The difference between these states can be compared to being conscious versus running on automatic pilot, and much of mindfulness practice involves noticing how often we are engaged in this automatic-pilot mode, and consciously bringing our awareness back into the moment. Mindfulness is not so much an end in itself but a way in which we can wake up to this rich, mysterious and ever-changing process of life.

WHAT ARE THE BENEFITS?

The state of mindfulness can be hard to describe and there is really no substitute for actually experiencing it. Through the practice, however, people often notice feeling more ease and openness and a sense of heightened awareness. It can help us to recognise the habits and patterns of the mind and give us a sense of control or choice, not habitually becoming caught up in the struggles or patterns that may cause stress or anxiety. People also report greater inner strength, contentment and improvements in relationships. There is now a significant body of scientific research on the practice of mindfulness and its beneficial effects on reducing stress, anxiety, depression and improving health and well-being.

WHAT ARE THE ORIGINS?

The practice of mindfulness goes back thousands of years, and despite being most strongly associated with Buddhism, it shows up within nearly all other religions and spiritual traditions. More recently there has been an explosion of interest in mindfulness as a secular practice, without the religious associations. There are many books and experiential courses on mindfulness and these could be a valuable addition to what appears in this book in developing a deeper understanding of the practice.

IS MINDFULNESS THE SAME AS MEDITATION?

This is a common question. People often use the word meditation to refer to a particular practice, such as sitting or lying down and bringing the awareness to the breath or some other aspect of experience. Mindfulness, however, can be understood as an orientation towards our experience and can be practised in any situation in daily life, including while eating, washing the dishes, walking the dog or hanging out the laundry. Remembering to be mindful and stepping out of automatic pilot can be challenging, and the practice of mediation can be a helpful way to develop and strengthen this ability.

I think it is also helpful to notice if we get caught up in judging certain states or experiences as better than others. We can easily give ourselves a hard time for not being 'mindful enough', and in this way our relationship to meditation or mindfulness practice can be striving and self-critical. Finding a balance of having the intention to be awake to the moment and applying the right amount of effort towards this, while having acceptance and self-compassion, can be an ongoing dance.

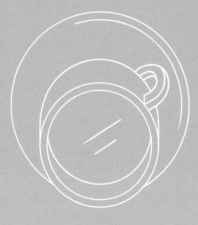

'Drink your tea slowly
and reverently, as if it is
the axis on which the
whole earth revolves –
slowly, evenly, without
rushing toward the
future; live the actual
moment. Only this
moment is life.'

THICH NHAT HANH

SOME COMMON
MISCONCEPTIONS ABOUT
MINDFULNESS AND MEDITATION

Mindfulness and mediation are about emptying the mind of thoughts

Many people I have talked to say that mindfulness and meditation are not for them, as they have either tried it and failed or think they are not capable of it. When I explore this with them it usually comes down to them believing that meditation is about not having any thoughts, and when they try this they very soon find it is an impossible task. Mindfulness is not so much about getting rid of thoughts but relating to them differently; it is allowing them to come and go without getting caught up in them, while making more space for other aspects of our experience.

Mindfulness is about positive thinking

Mindfulness is not about trying to have positive thoughts, or even trying not to have negative thoughts. When people start practising they soon realise that they have little control over the thoughts that come to their mind. Through mindfulness we can learn to relate differently to our thoughts, observing them with awareness, not taking them too seriously or feeling them to be always true. This relationship can help us untangle from our thoughts without judging them or trying to make them go away.

Mindfulness is just for New Agers and hippies

Mindfulness now has a significant scientific evidence base and it is being used in numerous settings, including hospitals, schools, businesses, universities and prisons. With a growing interest, perhaps resulting from the stresses of modern life and the rigorous research on their benefits, mindfulness-based approaches seem to have transcended the label of alternative therapies.

Mindfulness will make all my problems go away

Difficulty and pain seem to be an inherent part of life, and no matter what we do we will experience difficulties, such as ill health, the loss of loved ones, or financial challenges. Mindfulness does not eliminate or fix all of our worldly problems, but it may help us relate differently to difficulties as they inevitably arise in our lives.

Mindfulness makes a lot of sense and is a great idea

Unfortunately just reading books and understanding the concept of mindfulness will do very little other than give us something else to talk about. The cultivation of mindfulness is an experiential endeavour, it takes time and commitment to experience what it really has to offer and there are no quick fixes or magic wands.

ATTITUDES THAT SUPPORT US IN MINDFULNESS

The cultivation of mindful awareness is a gradual and subtle process and one that is not easily measured. Mindfulness in essence is a state of awareness and can only be experienced in any given moment. However, there are certain shifts in attitude and perspective that may begin to develop and in return support this process. Jon Kabat-Zinn, one of the pioneers in bringing mindfulness practice to the Western world, describes a number of attitudes that he sees as fundamental in supporting mindful awareness.

1. NON-JUDGEMENT

It is natural that we make judgements about ourselves and the world around us. With mindfulness we can begin to become aware of this process of 'judging mind' and rather than becoming caught up or further fuelling these judgements, instead we take on the role of impartial observer. We can practise this as we walk, first by noticing how judgement shows up for us, maybe how fit we feel or if we find what we see around us pleasant or not, if there are 'too many' other people on our walk, etc. These kinds of judgements are natural, so there is no need to further judge yourself for having them; simply notice them. The act of awareness in itself gives us space and freedom. By noticing and letting go of judgement we allow ourselves to experience fully the moment as it actually is.

2. PATIENCE

An attitude of patience helps us be with each moment as it arrives rather than trying to rush through certain moments that we consider to be less important in order to get to better ones. We allow things to unfold in their own time and give our attention to each moment. When out on a walk in the mountains, we may be rushing to get to the top as we think the view will be better. The act of rushing will not make the view any better when we get there, and in the process it prevents us from appreciating what is available to us each step of the way. The attitude of patience can also be turned towards ourselves and our mindfulness practice, allowing ourselves to be who and where we are. When out walking we may notice when we become impatient and how this makes us feel. If we observe nature it does not seem to be in a rush; it has its own natural rhythms with day and night and the seasons. Perhaps observing this can support us in developing our own patience.

3. BEGINNER'S MIND

The attitude of beginner's mind is one of curiosity towards our experience, trying to see things with fresh eyes as they really are in the moment rather than letting our beliefs, opinions and judgements shape our experience. It is a reminder that each moment is unique. We allow things to be alive, to change, to be fresh in each moment. We are open to the extraordinariness of life rather than sinking into the ruts of our knowledge or expertise. You can explore bringing this attitude of beginner's mind to people, places and the things you see around you, and notice how this may change your experience of them. The same walk can be different every time if we are open in this way.

4. TRUST

The practice of mindfulness is not about trying to become a 'better' person, or more like somebody else, but rather to become more fully who we already are. An attitude of trust in our own experience, intuition, goodness and wisdom supports us in this, regardless of whether we have made mistakes. It also emphasises taking on responsibility for our own well-being; only we can live our own lives.

5. NON-STRIVING

The practice of mindfulness is not goal-oriented, although at first this may seem counterintuitive. The process is not one of trying to achieve some other state or of changing ourselves, but of letting go of this struggle. Paradoxically this shift in orientation seems to allow for changes to happen but not through striving. Striving to make our experience or ourselves different or better often causes us struggle and frustration. A helpful analogy with mindfulness is that the best way of getting from A to B is to first be fully with A.

6. ACCEPTANCE

The attitude of acceptance is not a resignation but the ability to be with the reality of our experience in the moment, rather than getting caught up in the struggle, tension and mental effort of wanting things to be different, or denying how they are. Acceptance allows us to settle into the moment and be with what is. This does not mean we have to be passive or just submit to things; we can still make decisions, take action or make changes, but they come from a place of seeing how things really are.

When out walking, if it begins to rain we may habitually hunch our shoulders, speed up and focus on getting to a dry, warm place out of the 'unpleasant' rain. In contrast, how might it be to accept that it is raining and to experience it for what it is, straighten up, allow the raindrops to fall on us, feel the sensation of the coolness of the water on our skin and hear the sound of raindrops? We may find that this radically changes our experience and, rather than resisting the situation, we accept, embrace and even enjoy it.

7. LETTING GO

We can expend a great deal of mental effort holding on to or attaching ourselves to things, whether these are our opinions, ideas, desires, situations or events, or people that we want or don't want in our lives. Letting go involves recognising when the mind is gripping or tightening around these things and intentionally allowing ourselves to put them aside.

The seven attitudes described here have a lot of crossover and are mutually supportive. Imagine them as the fertile soil from which mindfulness can grow and in turn mindfulness will help to deepen these attitudes.

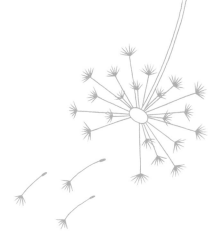

WALKING MEDITATION

Walking meditation has a long tradition within Buddhist practice as a way to developing mindfulness and is now included in mindfulness-based programmes used across settings, from reduction of stress and depression, to organisational psychology, schools and prisons.

The essence of the practice is to use the sensations that arise in the feet as we walk slowly as a place to focus attention, very much like the breath is often used in sitting meditation practice. This moment-by-moment attention to the sensations of present moment allows awareness to become more stable and offers a place to return to when we notice the mind is drawn away.

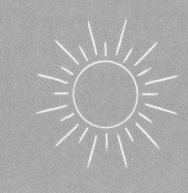

SOME OF THE BENEFITS OF
SUCH A PRACTICE INCLUDE:

- Focus and stability of awareness

- Familiarity with the patterns of the mind and what it gets involved with

- The opportunity to practice returning attention to the present moment

- Sensitivity to physical sensations in the body

PRACTICE:
WALKING MEDITATION

Ideally find a quiet place where you will not be disturbed. It can be indoors or outdoors and you might like to remove your shoes. Find two points on the ground around 10m (33/4ft) apart and stand on one of the points. When you are ready, bring your attention to the sensations of your body in this standing position. Allow the body to be upright and dignified, with the eyes looking ahead. As best you can, let go of any tension in the body and allow the breath to move freely. Then guide your awareness down through the body into the soles of your feet and notice the sensations of contact with the ground. You may want to experiment with gently rocking forwards and backwards or side to side and, as you do so, really notice how the shifting of your weight impacts the sensations in your feet. Now, very slowly, peel one foot from the ground, raise and slowly place it in front of you. It can be helpful to take small steps with the toe pointed slightly outwards to

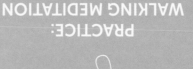

maintain balance. Track the sensations you feel in the soles of your feet through this process. Now lift and place the other foot slowly enough that you can focus in detail on the sensations.

Repeat this movement until you reach the second point. It can be helpful to come back to standing still for a while before turning and walking back. During this practice the mind will undoubtedly wander off into all kinds of places and this is not wrong. In fact, it is an essential part of the practice, as it allows us to practise noticing these movements of the mind, and purposefully to return the awareness to the moment-by-moment sensations in the soles of your feet. Each time you notice the mind is no longer present, simply come to stillness and, with an attitude of patience and acceptance, return the awareness and begin again.

PRACTICE:
COUNTING STEPS

A method that you may find helpful for keeping your attention focussed is to count in your head each time you place a foot down. When you reach ten you can start again at one. If you notice your mind has wandered and is no longer present with the sensations in the feet, you can pause, congratulate yourself for noticing a wandering mind, and begin again at one. If you choose to use this method of counting it is important to make the counting as subtle as possible so that your attention is still with the sensations in the feet and not just with the mental process of counting. Stay really attentive to the sensations as the foot comes to the floor, and only when the foot is still very gently make a mental note 'one', and so on.

PRACTICE: BROADENING
THE FIELD OF AWARENESS

For this walking meditation practice, rather than just focussing in a narrow way on the sensations in the feet, the awareness is expanded so that it takes in the whole body as it moves. Through these different practices we begin to notice that awareness is a flexible faculty and can be shifted from object to object as well as broadened and narrowed. It can be helpful to start with a more focussed practice, such as the one described above, to gather and focus the awareness before broadening it to take in the whole body, noticing the different sensations that arise and pass away as the body moves. You may also want to experiment with speed, noticing what happens to the awareness as you speed up or slow down.

Beyond the body, the awareness can be broadened into what you can see, hear and smell as you walk, noticing how the environment around you is sensed by your body, such as the warmth of the sun or wind against the skin, or the sounds of cars, birds or the sea.

'The mind can go in a thousand directions, but on this beautiful path, I walk in peace. With each step, the wind blows. With each step, a flower blooms.'

THICH NHAT HANH

THE BREATH

The breath can be a helpful companion in the development of mindful awareness by stabilising our attention, and it has been used in this way for thousands of years and across numerous meditative traditions.

As long as you are alive there is always breath and it is happening right now, moment by moment. By turning our attention to the direct physical sensations of the breath we can encourage our awareness to form a link with the present moment. Even if this doesn't last for long there is always a new breath to come back to whenever the mind whisks us off into the past or future. It is something we can repeatedly return to, to re-centre ourselves.

The breath also changes as a result of our current physical and mental state and can be an indicator to us of what we are experiencing. We might hold our breath when we feel tense or anxious, and use slow, soft breaths when we are calm. You might explore this for yourself and see what your breath tells you about your inner world throughout the day.

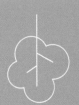

PRACTICE:
BREATHING

When out on a walk, come to a standing position somewhere you feel comfortable and where you will not feel self-conscious. Find a position where the body can relax, yet remain upright, with a feeling of openness and space around your chest, and with your arms resting by your sides. Close your eyes or lower your gaze so that you can turn your attention inwards. Take a moment to notice how the body feels in this moment, the physical sensations of your posture and the sensation of your feet meeting the ground. When ready, turn your attention towards the sensations of breathing. Be curious. Where can you feel movements of the air from the breath: the air entering your nose or against the back of your throat; the rising and falling of your chest or the movements in your abdomen. It is important actually to focus on the direct physical sensation rather than thinking about or visualising the breath – there is an important difference. Settle on the feeling of the breath in one place and follow the sensations of each in-breath and each out-breath moment by moment. Sooner or later the mind may wander off, become caught up in a chain of thoughts, a memory or whatever. This is totally natural. It is what minds do and the task is simply to come back to the sensation of the breath each time this happens. After a while, allow your awareness to expand into the feeling of your whole body as it stands and breathes, feeling the rising and falling of your chest and shoulders, noticing your feet against the floor and the edges of your body where it comes into contact with the world around it. Gently open your eyes and as you continue to walk see if you can stay in touch with any awareness or focus you may have touched into, knowing that at any time you can come back to the feeling of your breath to anchor and stabilise your awareness.

NO DESTINATION

Often when we walk, even if it is not obvious to us, our destination or what that destination will involve is at the forefront of our minds. We may be walking to the shops, thinking what we are going to buy, or walking to a meeting and rehearsing what we will say, or even when walking for recreation we may be subtly focusing on trying to reach our destination, whether it is the top of a mountain or a waterfall.

Similar patterns of being pulled forward by the mind will likely show up at other times in daily life, and walking can be a good place to notice and become familiar with it. How does it feel? Is it possible to bring our attention to where our mind is occupied and to deliberately let go of the destination, to walk for each step, for each sound, and for each sight as we experience them moment by moment?

The process is a dynamic one and we may find moments of being very aware and present and then being drawn back to the patterns of thinking, planning, remembering or wherever the mind is taking us. It is helpful to be playful and easy around this process, not trying to force anything, but rather to relax into our experience.

'Take my hand.
We will walk. We
will only walk. We
will enjoy our walk
without thinking of
arriving anywhere.'

THICH NHAT HANH

SLOWING DOWN

There appears to be reciprocal connections between the way we hold and move our bodies and how we feel, our internal world and mood. This is something we can readily experience first-hand. When you are feeling tired or fed up, just try bringing your awareness to your posture. Are you upright and alert in the body or perhaps slightly hunched, with heaviness in the neck and shoulders? If this is the case, by the action of bringing more uprightness to the body and looking around, you may notice a shift in how you feel. And smiling, even if forced at first, naturally seems to lift our mood.

How we walk can also reveal connections between mind and body. If our mind is occupied with where we are going, or if we are in a conversation, we may find

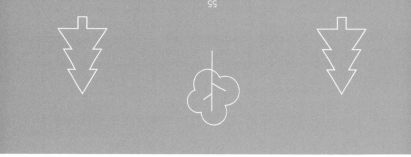

ourselves walking faster, even hurrying. If we deliberately slow down this can have an effect on the activity of the mind. Slowing down can be the physical embodiment of letting go of urgency, of trying to get somewhere else, of stepping ahead of where we actually are.

Experimenting with the speed of how we walk and how this affects our awareness can be an insightful exercise and, when walking mindfully and really paying attention to what is around you, you may naturally find yourself walking more slowly than usual.

Stopping and taking some time to be still can be a continuation of this and I will talk a little more about building mindful pauses into walks later in the book (see page 110).

Of all the ways
we humans move,
walking has to be
the best way of
going slowly.

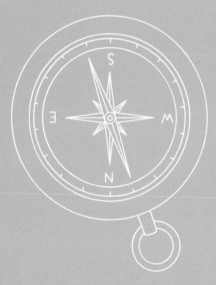

SPEEDING UP

Although it can be helpful, we do not have to be slow to be mindful.

SOMETIMES THE BODY FEELS LIKE IT NEEDS TO MOVE, RUN, OR DANCE TO BE EXERTED

We often find pleasure and exhilaration in this movement. More vigorous movement can lead to clear changes in the body and bringing awareness into these physical sensations is a way we can stay present in the body. We can attend to the feeling of the depth and rate of the breath, the heartbeat, the blood flowing through the body and the release of endorphins, perhaps feeling more alive and appreciative of the simple joy of movement.

WALKING AND SILENCE

Going for a walk with other people can be an enjoyable and connecting experience, catching up, joking, sharing stories and observations. Walking often facilitates and eases the conversation. We can drop in and out, pausing to appreciate what is around. Talking, however, can also keep us quite engaged with our thoughts, whether this is reflecting on what the other person has just said, or thinking about what our response will be. It may conjure up memories, images and ideas.

With all this going on, we may find we tend to notice less of what is going on around us or in our own bodies and be less connected to the present moment. When it comes to mindfulness or mindful walking, times of silence can be highly supportive.

For many of the practices outlined in this book I would recommend trying them in silence. You may know people who are quite happy to drop into silence when sharing company on a walk, otherwise you can arrange ways of supporting this. When I lead mindful group walks we deliberately space ourselves out while walking and come together to share our experiences. Paradoxically something that people nearly always comment on is how they feel more connection to others in the group through this way of walking.

Walking alone, if you feel confident and safe to do so, is also a good option for a mindful walk.

Some of my richest experiences of walking have been when I've headed out into the mountains for a few days alone. Walking alone gives me the feeling of having the time to catch up with a good friend, following my own speed and intuitions, pausing to take in what is around me whenever I feel like. In company there is pleasure in the sharing of experience, we may sometimes comment on the beauty of what we notice around us. Alone, however, I have found these experiences are no less special for the lack of sharing. In your own company there is still a relationship and a sharing, albeit with yourself, and time alone seems to deepen and enrich this relationship.

SILENCE BECOMES LIKE A CONTAINER FOR OUR AWARENESS, HELPING US TO STAY IN TOUCH WITH THE PRESENT MOMENT

STOPPING IN YOUR TRACKS

It can be a fruitful practice to notice where your mind goes when you are walking, seeing how one thought leads to another; how images, memories, judgements and feelings arise and pass away. Maybe we feel a sense of hunger and the mind fixates on reaching a place to stop for food, imagining what we will eat; or if we are near the end of a walk, the mind is already at the car or back home planning our next task. This mind wandering is a natural part of life, but awareness of it allows us the space to choose whether to continue entertaining the thoughts or place our awareness elsewhere for a while.

While walking, the act of stopping can help us settle the mind and set the intention to re-centre ourselves. It can be useful to take a moment to close your eyes, feel the sensations of your feet against the ground and follow a few breaths. You might ask yourself: 'Do I really need to give my attention to whatever the mind was involved with right now?' Perhaps you do or perhaps you can let go of whatever it is and come back to being with the walking. This regular checking in is not only a valuable practice in returning awareness to the present moment, but it is also a way of becoming more familiar with the patterns of the mind and the places it keeps taking us.

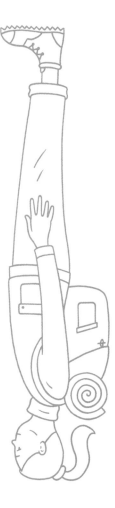

and open at the same time.
dignified quality that is relaxed
embodies an upright, alert and
intention. The standing mountain
the posture can help set this
back into the moment, adjusting
When pausing to guide awareness

with you as you walk.
or clarity from taking this pause
to bring the awareness, presence
begin to walk again, you are able
look around, see whether, as you
feel you can open your eyes and
tiring and discouraging. Once you
into a battle with it tends to be
activity of the mind or entering
and self-compassion. Judging the
it, along with requiring intention
and effort, also requires patience
its own, and learning to work with
mind can appear to have a life of
mind's incessant activity. The
a sense of humour around the
this process and even to develop
It is important to be gentle in

PRACTICE: PAUSING

When you notice that the mind is not present.

5. Continue to walk, seeing if you can bring with you any groundedness and presence from this practice.

4. Open your eyes and notice what you see around you while still holding an awareness of the physical presence of the body.

1. Pause and come to a comfortable, relaxed position with your eyes closed or your gaze lowered.

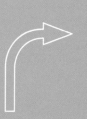

2. Ask: 'Do I need to entertain these thoughts right now?' If not, allow yourself to let them go.

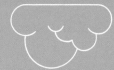

3. Bring your awareness into the body, feeling the sensations of your feet against the ground and the breath as it enters and leaves.

ATTENDING TO THE SENSES

When we walk, we go out into the world and we meet this world through our sense of touch, sight, sound, smell and taste. Giving more attention to what we notice though our senses can help us become more present.

Although this may sound simple, as humans we have an amazing capacity for thinking, interpreting, remembering and projecting into the future. This ability to be highly adaptive helps us to survive in the world, but on the flip side it can quickly take us away from our direct experience, using up our limited capacity for attention and leaving little space for awareness of the richness that is available to our senses from moment to moment. Being more fully aware of our senses does not mean we will stop thinking, but it can give us more space and freedom around the thoughts akin to turning down the volume on a radio.

Walking and being out in the natural world can be a great opportunity to explore this. It can be helpful to be playful in this experience and enter with a mind of curiosity, as if you are a child or a being from another planet

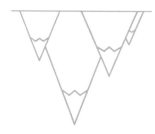

experiencing the world for the first time, letting go a little of 'already knowing' and seeing the world with fresh eyes. If we think we know something, then our attention tends to move on. We see a tree or a flower; our mind labels it, 'oak tree', we have a concept, a name, a familiarity, and our interest may be lost, our mind has other things to 'do'. With an attitude of curiosity, of not knowing, we can stay longer with the actual direct and unique experience of that tree, the shapes, colours, patterns, movements, sounds and smells. The filters of our conceptual mind may drop away and we wake up to an 'aliveness', the space where our senses meet the world directly, moment by moment.

The following pages outline some practices that can help us tune into our senses and explore the landscape of our awareness.

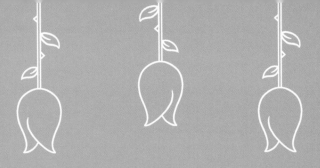

Don't forget
to stop and smell
the roses.

PHYSICAL SENSATION

Awareness of the physical body is a valuable gateway into the present moment and it has been used extensively in meditative practices and traditions. From attending to the breath during sitting meditation, the feeling of the feet against the ground in walking meditation, the sensations of the body in movement and breath in mindful yoga practice, Qigong and Tai Chi, physical sensations are always happening in the present. Tuning into them can anchor our awareness and help us feel more embodied. As well as the meditative traditions above, we can do this while walking and interacting with the natural world around us. This is great news, if, like me, you are naturally drawn to the outdoors.

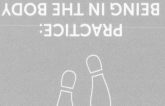

PRACTICE:
BEING IN THE BODY

Find a place where you are unlikely to be disturbed or feel self-conscious. This could be your back garden or a quiet area of woodland. First, find a seat or stand and close your eyes. Take some time to notice the physical sensations of your body making contact with the ground and really let your awareness fully inhabit these sensations, feeling them from the inside, not just thinking about them. Allow your awareness to settle and rest for a while in these sensations. When you are ready, allow your awareness to expand into the whole body. Notice the position of your body, the movements it makes as it draws in air and expels it with each breath, even notice your heart beating. After a while, guide your awareness to the sensations of contact between your body and the environment around you: the feeling of the wind against your skin, the coolness of the air or the warmth from the sun. During the practice you will almost undoubtedly find that the mind becomes involved or that you have been carried away on a particular train of thought. This is totally natural and the act of noticing is an important step in being able to come back. However many times this happens, without judging yourself, simply return the awareness to the sensations in the body.

When you feel ready you can open your eyes, noticing what happens as you do this. Begin to explore the environment around you through your sense of touch and physical sensation. The more you can be curious and open to this, the easier it will be to immerse yourself in the experience. As far as possible, suspend judgement of yourself or the practice. You may want to lie in the grass, explore the texture of tree bark with your fingers, or the feeling of leaves against the skin, the direct sensation of wind or sunlight on the body. You can do this with your eyes open or closed. Notice judgements from the mind or impulses to move on and see these just as mental events, not necessarily holding any truth, but drawing us away from the richness of our experience in the moment.

You can tune into this sense of the body at any time during the day in order to stabilise the awareness and return to the present.

SIGHT

For many of us sight is our most dominant sense, and yet when we begin to look in an active sense it can become apparent how much is going on that we usually miss: things that have been accessible to us for years but that we walk past without noticing. There is so much to notice when we are out walking and, by practising bringing a greater awareness to this sense, we can become more open and attentive to the world around us. Young children naturally seem to be more engaged in the present moment, and much of this is probably because experiences are new to them. Trying to see as if we are looking through the eyes of a child might be a helpful analogy for this practice, letting go of some of our knowing, as if we are seeing things for the first time.

'The real voyage of discovery consists not in seeking new landscapes but in having new eyes.'

MARCEL PROUST

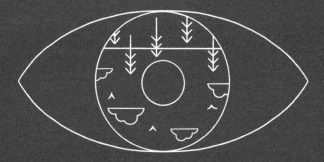

PRACTICE: SEEING

Stand or sit for a while with your eyes closed and become aware of the feeling of your body, how it makes contact with the ground, the sensations of breathing. Allow yourself to arrive into this moment, letting go as best you can of any thoughts. When you are ready, open your eyes and find a place on the ground in front of you to focus your gaze. See if it is possible to bring an attitude of freshness and novelty to this faculty of sight. Allow yourself to absorb what you can see, the colours, shapes and movements. You may notice that your mind begins to assign labels, such as 'grass', or 'twig' or 'dead leaf'. If you notice this, see if you can let go of the labels and come back to your direct experience of what you are seeing. Take some time to move your gaze around and take in more of your visual field, bringing the same attitude of curious interest to what you see. You might want to pick up an object and examine it in real detail, or walk around and explore your surroundings. Getting down low to the ground can enable you to see the reflection on a water droplet, the patterns on a beetle's back or the intricacy of a moss or lichen. Explore the world from all angles, from the micro to the macro.

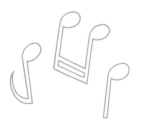

SOUND

The vibrations of the world around us, coming into contact with our eardrums and being interpreted by the brain, give us a rich vault of information and experience. It allows for language, the sharing of our personal worlds, signals danger, music, birdsong and the sound of traffic, to name just a few. Sounds are constantly in flux, arising into our awareness and fading away; they are like a mirror reflecting the ever-changing, impermanent nature of our experience. Sounds also give rise to images, labels and judgements as the mind interprets them. We can use the field of sound as a gateway into the ever-changing moment, letting go of concepts and returning to direct experience.

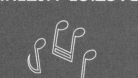

PRACTICE: LISTENING

Begin this practice by taking a few moments to come to stillness and connect with the physical sense of the body being here in this moment. Closing your eyes can be helpful for this practice, so you may want to find a place to sit. When you feel ready, shift your attention to what you can hear, to the world of sound.

Notice the different sounds that enter your awareness as you listen; some may be distant sounds while some may be close. As far as possible stay with the direct experience of the sounds, noticing their qualities, the pitch tone, duration and volume. You do not need to be active in this process. See if you can just allow sounds to come to you as if you are recording them. If you notice that your mind is beginning to label the sounds, as best you can, let go of this and bring your awareness back to the direct experience of the sounds themselves, moment by moment. You may even notice the silence between sounds, like a field into which each sound emerges. At a certain point you can open your eyes, seeing whether you can remain focussed on what you can hear.

Take a walk and notice how the sounds come and go or shift; perhaps you can hear the sound of your feet against the ground, the sound of the wind, of traffic, or of water. Some sounds may appear pleasant – birds singing, a trickling stream – and some perhaps less pleasant, such as car horns or shouting. Be curious about what pleasant, unpleasant or neutral sounds feel like; is it possible to be open to all these sounds, not allowing oneself to be caught up in judgement, simply allowing them to arise, linger and pass away?

SMELL

Our sense of smell is perhaps more subtle than the other senses. We may only pay attention to it if something has a particularly strong smell, either pleasant or unpleasant. Like the other senses, however, as we deliberately attend to smell we find that there may be more going on than we are typically aware of. Smell also has a particularly strong connection with memory, and certain scents can bring back images and feelings from our past. When out walking, deliberately tuning into this sense provides another way to be more directly in contact with the world around you and your experience in the moment.

PRACTICE: SMELL

Find a place where you are not likely to be disturbed and first take some time to guide your awareness to your present-moment experience, feeling your body and breath, and as best you can, letting go of other thoughts or concerns you may be holding. As you breathe, allow your awareness to rest with the air as it enters the nostrils. Can you detect any scent in the air? If so, notice its qualities. Is it sweet, tangy, fresh, floral, musty or woody? When ready, open your eyes and begin to explore the world around you. Explore picking things up or getting down close and fully immerse yourself in the sense of smell, breathing in the flavours of dead leaves, flowers or the bark of a tree. If you notice images or memories arising in your mind as you do this, allow space for these too. You may also notice the minds reaction or commentary to the practice through thoughts, feelings and judgments. Perhaps pleasure, delight or curiosity or aversion, boredom or distraction. There is no right or wrong just notice what interest what shows up. Take as long as you like to explore this sense, and your mind and body's reactions to the practice, allowing curiosity through the process. See if you can transfer this curiosity and awareness to your everyday walks.

WALKING WITH OPEN AWARENESS

In the previous practices we have been cultivating awareness of the individual senses. Through doing this practice we discover a surprising amount of detail and richness that often goes unnoticed. These practices also help develop our ability to place and move our attention voluntarily, rather than letting the mind flit from one thing to another of its own accord.

As well as directing awareness to a particular aspect of experience, such as what we see or hear, it is possible to hold a more open, undirected, or 'choiceless awareness', while at the same time remaining present. In this way, as we walk we can be open to all of our senses, allowing in whatever comes to us, the sounds, sights, sensations and smells, moment by moment, taking in the full tapestry of our experience. This awareness can lead to a sense of ease and openness as we walk.

PRACTICE: WALKING WITH AWARENESS

As you walk, allow yourself to take in what you see, hear, smell and feel. You may notice at times that a particular object of awareness, such as a sight or sound may draw you in. This is fine and you can let this catch your attention before allowing your awareness to expand again. Thoughts and feelings may come and go and these are just another aspect of your experience; see if you can hold them lightly. If you become deeply involved in a chain of thoughts, and are no longer aware in the present moment, then bring your awareness back to a couple of breaths, or the sensation of your feet against the ground, before once again broadening the awareness. It can take practice to work with the awareness in this way so don't worry if it does not make sense immediately. It is helpful to practice in a way that is gentle, so don't try and force anything; always hold an attitude of curiosity, ease and acceptance.

We can also be playful and curious as to how we relate to ourselves within this. Often we may have a sense of an identity looking out, hearing sounds that are coming from outside of us and touching a world separate to us. Although on one level this may seem true, it can be interesting to explore the possibility of inhabiting the broader field of our awareness, allowing a softening of the boundaries between 'me' and 'out there'.

CHALLENGING WALKS

Sometimes walking may be difficult or even unpleasant. We may be tired, challenged by a steep hill, our feet may hurt or we might get caught in a downpour. Perhaps we are on a stunning walk but the path is crowded with other people spoiling our peace and solitude. Situations like these can be opportunities to learn something about how we relate to, and even participate in, 'unpleasant experiences'. As well as perhaps enriching our experience of walking, this learning can be translated to many other situations in our lives.

First, we can begin to notice what is actually going on in our experience. Often we attribute our difficulties to something outside of ourselves, such as the steep hill, or the rain, or the crowds, so it is helpful to come back into what is actually happening. We can notice the sensations we are experiencing, like tired legs, deep breathing, fast heartbeat, or the feel of the rain on our skin, or the sight and sound of others around us. These direct experiences are often not unpleasant in themselves and the challenge comes in the form of our thoughts or judgements about them: for example, 'This hill is too long', 'I am tired', or 'I am going to get wet and cold, I wish it wasn't raining', or 'It is a lovely day but I wish all these people weren't here'. It is often this level of interpretation or judgement of our experience that causes us to suffer; the resistance to what is and the desire for it to be different. We may not be able to change the situation we are in but we can learn to respond differently.

PRACTICE: UNPLEASANT EXPERIENCES

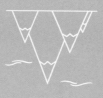

When you notice an unpleasant experience while walking use this as a wake-up call to what is really happening for you and become curious.

1. Notice what your direct experiences are in the body. Notice what you can see or hear around you.

2. How are you interpreting these experiences? Do you feel any resistance to your experience or judgements?

3. As best as you can, accept and let go of these. There is no need to judge yourself for having judgements these are natural.

4. Come back to the direct experience and see if you can accept it and let it be just as it is. Take one step at a time, one breath at a time.

OUR PLACE IN THE NATURAL WORLD

Walking can be a reminder of the wider natural world around us and the interconnected cycles of life that support our existence. This is perhaps more important now than ever with changing lifestyles and environmental challenges. Many jobs are now based indoors and developments in technology and entertainment mean we spend more time in front of screens. We no longer need to go outside to hunt, or put our hands in the soil to grow food. It all appears for us packaged on supermarket shelves and most of us are far removed from the processes of growth and the life and death that bought it there.

There is growing concern that this alienation from the natural world and its systems, especially for children, may not only impact our emotional and psychological well-being, but also how we relate to and treat our environment and planet. This recognition is leading to the creation of programmes to re-engage children with the natural world and to green up cities and community spaces. I don't believe we need to be in a remote wilderness to connect with the natural world. If we are open and aware, even in urban environments, a moment spent watching a bird, a tree pushing up through the pavement, or the smell of blossom in spring can link us to something beyond a purely human-concerned world.

The ideas that follow are ways of intentionally rekindling or deepening our connection to the natural world and our place within it.

SIMPLE IDEAS FOR FEELING
MORE CONNECTION WITH
THE NATURAL WORLD

Consciously make time

Even if it is just for five minutes each day, try and make a
habit of spending time with an awareness of the natural
world. This could be walking out into your garden in
the morning and listening to the birds, going for a short
mindful walk, or taking a lunch break outside and paying
attention to your surroundings and the life going on
around you.

Bring back reminders

If you visit a special place or have a connecting moment in
nature, take back a memento: a pebble, a feather, a piece
of driftwood or a shell. These can act as reminders, shrines
to the natural world inside your home.

Follow a natural impulse

When out walking, be curious and follow what draws
you in, perhaps getting up close with an intricate beetle,
following the sound of trickling water to a hidden stream,
or taking time to walk up to and examine a tree that
catches your eye, noticing what life is crawling over it or
growing on it.

See the world through different eyes

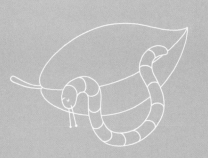

When out on a walk or in nature, try imagining experiencing the world as the animals and plants you see around you.

A bird circling, looking down for prey or gathering twigs for a nest to raise its young, a squirrel trying to collect enough nuts to bury for the winter, the long journey a caterpillar takes to reach the edge of a leaf. Taking in other views may lessen our own sense of self-importance and centrality to the world and make us more aware of the network of life unfolding around us.

Natural origins

Everything around us, including our food, furniture, homes, phones and cars, has origins in the natural world. It can be an interesting exercise to choose an item and reflect on how it came to be in its current form, running through all the stages, people and processes involved in the mind's eye, tracing it right back to its natural roots.

Changing perspective

In towns and cities we may view trees, plants and animals as pleasant features within an urban world. Experiment with flipping this perspective and seeing the buildings existing within a natural world, on top of soil, trees and plants bursting out between them.

Zoom in

While out walking, find a small area of ground, such as an old tree stump, an area of riverbank or patch of grass. Get up close and personal with this small patch, paying attention to what you can see: how the soil looks, what is decomposing, what is beginning to grow, what life is moving, insects, worms... Notice all that is going on, the cycles of life, just within this tiny part of the world.

See the diversity

Notice how many different plants and animals you can see; you do not need to know their names or try to remember them. Just become aware of their shapes, colours and movements, keeping the curiosity and interest alive.

Foraging

Foraging for food, whether that is berries, mushrooms, nuts or plants, not only gets us out into nature but puts us back in touch with our place in the food chain. We take an active role rather than being an onlooker and we have to move and expend energy for the rewards of what we eat. (Note: it is important to know what you can and can't eat, as wild food can be poisonous.)

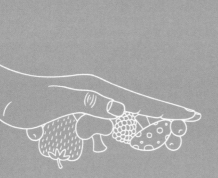

SEEING THROUGH SEPARATION

Contemplative wisdom traditions have long recognised our tendency as humans to relate to ourselves as somehow separate from the world around us and have developed practices to help us open to a deeper sense of our interconnectedness. The practices here offer a way of contemplating the natural cycles of life and our place within them, and will hopefully foster a deeper sense of connection and belonging within the natural world. They are based around the four symbolic elements of air, earth, water and fire. For the sake of these practices you do not need to hold any belief in the metaphysical importance of these elements. They simply offer a helpful framework through which to explore our connections with the world around us and see through a sense of separation.

These contemplations can be done anywhere, but if you can find a place out in the natural world, perhaps stopping during a walk in a quiet place and taking some time to sit, to look around you and to reflect, I think this can be even more effective.

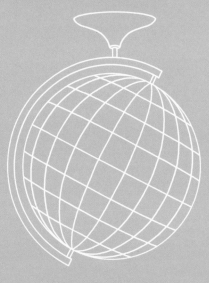

'When you realise
nothing is lacking,
the whole world
belongs to you.'

LAO TZU

PRACTICE: AIR

Begin this practice by bringing your awareness to the feeling of breathing, noticing the sensations of the air as it enters and leaves the body. This process of breathing began as soon as you entered the world and will continue until your last breath. It is a thread that connects every moment of your life. With each breath, you draw in vital oxygen, which is circulated to every cell in the body. Become aware of how totally dependent each of us is on this air all around us and the ability to keep breathing. Then begin to look around and become aware that you are surrounded by air. Feel it against your skin, the touch of the wind, how warm or cold it is. Become aware that it is this very air that you are breathing in that is sustaining your life. Then notice any other plants, trees or animals that you can see.

As you breathe, consider that this lungful of breath may have passed through and sustained countless other animals, plants and trees. Notice with each breath if you can let any sense of separation soften and fall away.

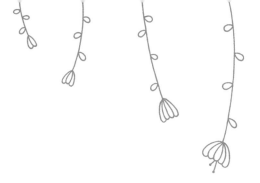

Contemplate how
each plant, each tree,
each living thing, is
also dependent on
this same air that is
passing between you
and within you.

Without food we
can survive for
weeks, but without
water only for a
matter of days.

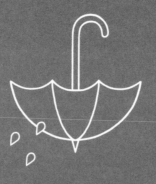

PRACTICE: WATER

Take some time to come to stillness and bring your awareness into the feeling of the body being in the moment; you may want to close your eyes to begin with. As you feel the presence of the body you might feel a sense of its solidity. However, around 50–65 per cent of our bodies is made up of water, and water is vital to survival.

Open your eyes, look and listen and take in the world around you. Notice where water is present: perhaps the clouds above you, the sound of a stream, and the drops of rain hanging on the trees or in the grass. Reflect on how this is the very same water that runs through our bodies, that we constantly replenish and excrete. It flows through us like it flows from the rivers into the sea, up into the sky and back down to earth. This same water is drawn up through the roots of trees and plants into their cells. Notice how every other living thing around you is also involved in this constant flow of the water cycle. How many other living things has the water in your glass passed through? We are made up of water, as are all other living things; it flows between us and the world around us. We are not separate from but part of this cycle.

PRACTICE: EARTH

Begin by bringing awareness into the feeling of your body as you stand or sit. Notice its weight, where its edges are, arriving at a sense of the physical solidity of this thing we call our body. Our bodies are a collection of cells (around 30 trillion), which themselves are made up of the elements that we and our mothers and fathers have absorbed from what we have eaten and drunk. Open your eyes and spend time looking around, feeling the ground. These same elements are present in everything you see around you: in other animals and plants, in the air, soil, rocks and oceans. When we die, like other animals and plants, our bodies will return to this cycle. Can you see leaves or twigs on the ground slowly decomposing back into the soil to be taken in again by other plants? We are part of this same cycle; our physical body is not separate from but part of an ever-changing system that includes and depends on the world all around us. The minerals in the soil become part of the vegetables we grow and these in turn become part of us when we eat them.

Spend some time contemplating these connections, walk around and explore the world, seeing the processes of growth and decay – the transfer of the elements.

What we regard as
our bones, blood,
organs and skin are
just a temporary
expression of this
interconnected
mineral world
represented here by
the earth element.

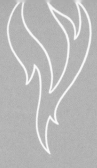

As we are
dependent on the
air we breathe, on
water and on the
mineral elements,
so, too, are we
dependent on heat
and energy.

PRACTICE: FIRE

The element fire can represent heat, energy and light. For this contemplation it can be good to go out on a sunny day or even build yourself a fire.

Not only do our bodies need to be above a certain temperature to survive, but without the energy from the sun, we could not survive, and neither could other animals or plants. Without the energy from the sun there would be no life on our planet. We can contemplate how the plant world captures this energy through photosynthesis, providing us with a food source as well as fuel for warmth and, more recently, all the developments of modern life. When we get in our cars it might not strike us that the sun we see through the windscreen is powering us, albeit through the process of photosynthesis and millions of years of its energy. The warmth of our own bodies from energy released through the food we eat has also come from this sun. Through contemplating this fire element we can see countless interconnections. Sit or stand for a while and feel the heat or coolness of the body, feel the warmth of the sun against your skin or the heat of a fire. When ready, open your eyes and look around you, noticing the connections between everything you see and this fire element.

CONNECT TO THE WORLD AROUND YOU

Contemplating the connections between ourselves and the world around us, and the cycles of life and the elements, may perhaps give us a different perspective on our lives: hopefully one in which we feel less separate from the natural world. This can add a new dimension to our time walking in nature.

IT MAY ALSO LEAD TO GREATER CONCERN & CUSTODIANSHIP FOR OUR ENVIRONMENT

'When we try to
pick out anything
by itself, we find
it hitched to
everything else in
the universe.'

JOHN MUIR

WALKING, APPRECIATION AND JOY

Walking and spending time out in the natural world offers numerous opportunities to tap into and cultivate positive emotions, such as appreciation, gratitude and joy. This can happen quite naturally when we witness a rare display of wildlife, the beauty of a spectacular view or sunset, or when we feel the warmth of the sun on our skin after a long winter. It can also arise in more modest moments if we pay attention. By bringing awareness to these feelings and experiences we can stay with them longer and cultivate our capacity to experience them more often.

'People usually consider
walking on water or in thin
air a miracle. But I think the
real miracle is not to walk
either on water or in thin
air, but to walk on earth.
Every day we are engaged
in a miracle which we don't
even recognise: a blue sky,
white clouds, green leaves,
the black, curious eyes of a
child – our own two eyes.
All is a miracle.'

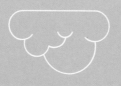

APPRECIATION AND GRATITUDE

These feelings can lift our mood and have a powerful effect on our sense of well-being. You can do a quick experiment of your own. First take a moment to notice how you are feeling right now. Spend some time paying attention to how your body feels, what is going on in your mind and your emotions. Now try and think of five things that you can be appreciative of and can be grateful for in your life right now. They don't have to be big things; it may just be the feeling of warmth of the cup of tea you are holding or seeing a bee going about its business moving from flower to flower. When you have noticed something, spend some time hanging out with it and really noticing how it feels before you move on to the next. The object of the exercise is to attend to the experience, not just to make a list. Once you have spent a few minutes, or however long you wish on this exercise, check in again with how you feel. There is no need to feel a certain way, just to notice what is true for you.

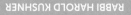

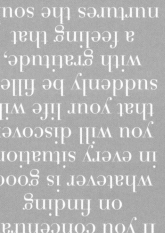

'If you concentrate on finding whatever is good in every situation, you will discover that your life will suddenly be filled with gratitude, a feeling that nurtures the soul.'

RABBI HAROLD KUSHNER

PRACTICE: APPRECIATION

Appreciate the world of the senses. The senses are our window into this world, and without them things would certainly be very different for us. It is pretty easy to take them for granted, unless perhaps we begin to lose them or they are threatened through age, illness or injury. Take a walk and spend some time intentionally noticing the amazing capacity of how our senses reveal the world to us. Immerse yourself in what you can see, hear, smell and feel, and notice if a sense of enjoyment and appreciation arises. This enjoyment is limitless and free – the light flickering on the water from the sun's reflection, or the movement of leaves as they rustle in the wind. Close your eyes and feel how your body is touched by the environment that surrounds it. Enjoy the sound of birds singing.

Where we place our attention shapes our minds and this shapes our lives. In this sense, if we deliberately take time to appreciate what is around us, then these feelings will naturally show up more in our lives. Each time you go out for a walk, why not take some time at the end to make a mental list of what you noticed or experienced that brought a sense of appreciation, connection, humour or interest?

Appreciate as you walk, your body goes through a complex sequence of movements, of fine balance and adjustment: the lungs work to bring in oxygen; the digestive system provides fuel and the heart beats to supply these vital ingredients to each cell. The body is constantly working for us in this way, and thankfully most of this happens without the need for our conscious effort. We may take this for granted, but spending some time contemplating and feeling gratitude for whatever our bodies still have the capacity to do for us is another way to open to more appreciation and joy in our lives. Can we relate to our body as if it is a dear friend, worthy of care and respect? How does it feel to hold this attitude?

PRACTICE: TAPPING INTO JOY WHILE WALKING

Walking can be a time to practise observing joy through the movement of the body, the greater depth of our breath and all that we see, hear, smell and feel around us.

1. As best you can, let go of any thoughts or concerns that you are holding, and gently guide your awareness to your present-moment experience.

2. Ask yourself: 'What joy might be available in this moment if I give it my attention?'

3. Without striving or trying to make your experience different simply notice what comes up for you. Is there any feeling of joy and how do you experience this in your body and mind? Is it related to something that you can see, hear or feel?

4. Allow yourself to spend time with these feelings for as long as they last, and when and if they go, just smile and carry on. There is no need to try and hold on to them. Every experience has a beginning and an end.

'The present
moment is filled
with joy and
happiness. If you
are attentive, you
will see it.'

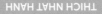

THICH NHAT HANH

THE SEASONS

Living a good few degrees north of the equator I have really grown to appreciate the changing seasons as the Earth tilts and orbits the sun.

IT IS ONE OF THE NATURAL RHYTHMS OF LIFE

The seasons mark the years that go by and give nature the opportunity to display in full colour its ever-changing aspect. Each season offers its own flavours, treats and feel, and by spending time outside and walking we can become tuned in to and appreciative of each one. Certainly sunshine seems to have an uplifting effect on most people's moods, but I fondly remember walking along a mountain ridge being battered by the wind and rain and my skin tingling with the cold. This in itself had its own beauty and unique expression of aliveness. The seasons provide an opportunity for noticing, for staying curious and engaged with the world around us, and help us to open up to the larger tapestry of the patterns of life that continue regardless of our everyday worries and concerns.

PAYING ATTENTION
TO THE SEASONS

Notice the plants and trees around you: when do they come into flower or leaf over the spring and summer, and when do they lose their leaves in the autumn? How do they respond to the seasons and the environment around them: the wind, the sun and the rain?

You can try the same with animals, being curious about what you can see or hear at different times of day and throughout the year.

When out walking pay attention to the position of the sun. Notice its arc traced through the sky as the world turns and how the shape of this arc and the position of the sun as it rises and sets change over the seasons.

Make an effort to get out at all times of year and in all types of weather to experience the seasons. Notice how streams, rivers and lakes change: sometimes bursting or gushing with water, and at other times almost dry.

Notice the feel or smell of the different seasons, the warmth or coolness, the humidity, the scent of blossom or the musty smell of a forest in autumn.

STILLNESS

Walking and movement can be a rich source of well-being, resilience and an avenue to explore and connect with the natural world around us. A number of traditions and cultures have also recognised the benefits of spending time in stillness out in the natural world as a way of connecting more deeply with our lives and the world around us: a way of gaining insights.

THERE IS SOMETHING IN THE QUALITY OF STILLNESS

In stillness there is no escape; we come up against the patterns of our mind without distraction and in this perhaps gain both insight and also learn to let go. Finding a place in the natural world just to be still can be an eye-opening experience when we begin to let go of the sense of having to do anything, to go somewhere else or to achieve something. It can also be a challenging practice, to step off the treadmill of our busy lives and, for a while, just be.

THAT RUNS COUNTER TO OUR HABITUAL TENDENCIES

We may encounter experiences such as resistance, boredom or restlessness. This in itself can be valuable if we are able to see these just as states of mind and allow them to come and go with acceptance. What learning might there be from simply sitting still in this world? Not learning in the sense of achieving, or gaining knowledge – for that it is better to read a book – but learning through letting go, tuning into our sensitivity, our raw aliveness which is so often hidden under the surface, submerged as we busy ourselves with activity.

PRACTICE: STILLNESS

This practice can be done for any length of time, from 30 minutes to a full day, witnessing sunrise to sunset. It is helpful, however, to set some boundaries ahead of time so that you can let go into the practice and not be distracted by needing to make decisions.

I think it is also helpful to approach this practice without goals or expectations, but simply with the intention to stay with the process, and be present to what unfolds. Find a place ideally in a natural setting, where you are unlikely to be disturbed. When you have chosen your spot, imagine a circle about 2m (6ft) in diameter around you; this will be your boundary for the time you have chosen. Within this space and over the time you have set, something will happen, your experience will change from moment to moment and there is no right or wrong to what unfolds. Try to stay with the process and be curious of what you notice.

This practice has the potential to conjure up powerful feelings, so it is important to be sensitive to your level of readiness, and whether it is a good time in your life.

If in doubt, start small and work from there. It can also be helpful to do this practice with others (but in separate places) or have a friend or therapist that you can share your experience with when you get back. Take enough warm clothes, water and food if you need to (sometimes people choose to fast to sharpen awareness).

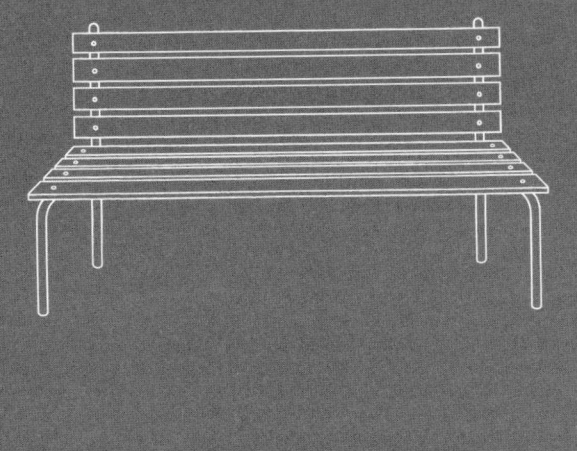

WALKING, CREATIVITY AND PERSPECTIVE

There is something about the act of walking that seems to provide a catalyst for creative thinking, perspective and reflection: the combination of its rhythm, the increased blood flow to the brain and the way it engages us bodily – and yet at the same time allows the mind freedom. This quality to walking has been recognised and appreciated across time and cultures, by philosophers, poets, and mystics including Nietzsche, Thoreau, Rousseau, Wordsworth and Gandhi, to name but a few. More recently research carried out at Stanford University in the United States suggests that walking indeed seems to increase creativity both during and shortly after the act.

As well as using walking as a way to cultivate mindfulness, it can be an opportunity to think creatively to generate ideas or gain perspective. When we walk we give ourselves physical distance from what we have been occupied with, whether this is our work, our domestic situation or perhaps even a relationship conflict or issue. This physical space seems to help us change perspective and the movement of the body allows the mind to move when otherwise we might feel blocked.

'All truly great
thoughts are
conceived by
walking.'

FRIEDRICH NIETZSCHE

PRACTICE:
WALKING TO REFLECT

Try this practice when you feel you could use some creative thinking time or to gain perspective. This could be regarding a particular challenge you are facing at work or at home, a conflict, or even if you have a life question or transition you would like to give time to.

First, try framing or articulating what it is that you hope to gain perspective or understanding about. You might phrase this as a specific question or it could be more open. Find a place to walk that is conducive to reflection. As you walk, allow the flow of thoughts to come and go naturally, moving at a speed that is in rhythm with this process, remaining aware of what comes up. Try not to become too fixated on finding a specific answer but be open to what emerges. You might want to take a journal to note down key ideas or themes. As best you can stay mindful in the process. Can you notice your reactions and feelings as thoughts arise? You can also pause from time to time to re-centre yourself and perhaps remind yourself of the intention or question you have.

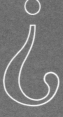

'Problems cannot
be solved at the
same level of
awareness that
created them.'

ALBERT EINSTEIN

TAKING A LONG WALK

Some of my fondest memories, of times when I have felt most alive and contented, are of long walking trips: the Himalayas, the Alps, the Scottish Highlands, and the Dolomites. The simplicity of just walking with no concerns but the basics of food and shelter. Moving through stunning wild landscapes, the body breathing deeply, the heart beating, and a genuine tiredness at the end of the day. Life becomes simple and yet at the same time it seems more fulfilling. All the things that we usually fill our lives wait thousands of footsteps away and are not missed. Our work becomes the filling of a bottle from a trickling mountain stream, our leisure is seeing sparkles of light dancing on the water, feeling its coolness on our hands and quenching a well-earned thirst.

The awareness naturally seems to become more heightened, the mind freed from the decisions and demands of life. In modern society, it is easy to get caught in the common dream that we must keep filling the holes within ourselves and our time with the next item or activity. Food, alcohol, drugs, TV, the Internet, shopping… the list goes on. Out on long walks in remote places, there is little temptation and there is no gap left by their absence, just some space for contentment and appreciation to show themselves.

To sit high up on a mountain path, the body rushing with endorphins, surrounded by sky, mountains, wild flowers and soaring birds, a sandwich packed for lunch, we realise that there is nothing else we need right now, there is nothing missing. These moments are certainly available to us in everyday life too but I believe that there is something about the cumulative effect of spending longer periods out walking that allows us to settle more deeply into such experiences.

There are many places in the world that provide excellent long walking opportunities, whether you choose to carry tents and camping gear, or to lighten your pack and walk from hut to hut. There are also many guided trips if you feel you lack the experience to go independently. Reading through guidebooks and magazines can be a good way to obtain inspiration and ideas.

The idea of walking for days on end may seem off-putting at first but I believe the rewards are well worth the effort and encourage you, if you are not hooked already, to give it a try!

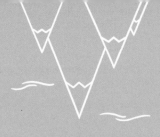

'Few places in this
world are more
dangerous than home.
Fear not, therefore,
to try the mountain
passes. They will kill
care, save you from
deadly apathy, set you
free, and call forth every
faculty into vigorous,
enthusiastic action.'

JOHN MUIR

The starry sky can
also provide an
interesting window
for an exploration
of our perception.

WALKING AT NIGHT

At night, the world takes on a different character. Things that seem familiar, predictable and safe to us during the day can shift dramatically with the absence of light and seem mysterious – even scary. Walking through a woodland perhaps epitomises this separation between night and day: the snapping of sticks underfoot or the gust of wind through the leaves meets heightened and more vigilant senses, as the unknown and unseen are colourfully filled by an active imagination. But this fear or tension is often not justified and, when the mind rests from its imaginings, we may settle into a different state. Our sharpened senses and the novelty of the experience draws us in and we perhaps feel more alive, more vital.

For me, one of the greatest treats of being out at night is a starry sky. Our daytime ceiling lifts and opens, and we see out into the vastness of space, the solar system, galaxy and the wider universe.

Looking out at the night sky might naturally leads to a change in perspective; the concerns of our lives, our own self-importance, are perhaps harder to take so seriously against the backdrop of a seemingly infinite universe. It can be humbling and probably a healthy experience if we allow ourselves the time to look out and wonder.

I remember the first time I felt I really looked out at the stars as a young adult; prior to that I had been looking up at the stars and seeing the constellations and planets with a mind accustomed to looking for patterns and meaning. That night I was sleeping out on a beach. It was clear, with no moon, and I began to focus on individual stars, reminding myself that each of these was a sun with its own planets, the larger ones closer and the smaller ones further away. After doing this for a while, something curious happened to my perception: the constellations dropped away, each star became unrelated to these purely conceptual patterns and the night sky took on a far more three-dimensional appearance. I had the feeling that I was really looking out into the universe in all directions rather than looking up at the sky. I still find I have the tendency to see the constellations when I look up and in a way I enjoy the familiarity with their place and movement during the night. Since that day I have also explored this other way of seeing, and it is a reminder to me of how our concepts play such a major role in shaping our perception of the world.

The Perseid
meteor shower

Each year the earth's orbit takes us through
a band of debris left by the Swift–Tuttle
comet and we experience a period of
meteor showers or shooting stars. This can
be a great time to go out for night walks
or to find a place to lie down and gaze up
at the night sky. The Perseids are visible for
up to a month, but the peak density falls
for a couple of days around mid-August.

WALKING IN LIFE

When life becomes busy or stressful it seems all too easy to let go of the things that are good for us, that help us to relax, maintain perspective and stay mentally and physically healthy. Perhaps we get caught in the pattern of thinking that we can only make time for ourselves once we have finished all the tasks on our list, or we just find ourselves doing it less and less until we get out of the habit.

Intentionally taking the time to walk can be an effective way of giving ourselves space as well as exercise, and paradoxically it may give us the sense of having more time. For example, we may feel really stressed or stuck on a particular issue at work, and the pressure of this may lead us to keep working over the lunch break to try to get it done. To leave the computer behind and get out and walk, even for ten minutes, might clear some space and, on returning to work, it could even help address the task at hand with new creativity or perspective. Ideas might come to us while we walk, our bodies will feel better, more awake, blood will flow to the brain – we will have respite from being hunched at a desk.

The following pages include some ideas for intentionally bringing more walking into our lives.

When you are at work, get into the habit of taking a short walk during lunch periods. See if you can make this a time and space where, rather than thinking of your work or task list for the afternoon, you practise being present in your experience and what is around you, perhaps trusting that connecting into this space in itself may bring what you need.

Each time you step outside, bring awareness to what you notice around you. How does the weather feel? Is it cold, with the wind against your skin or the touch of rain? Which flowers are out? What are the colours of the leaves on the trees? Just paying attention and noticing these things can naturally bring our awareness into the moment and puts us in touch with the ever-changing world around us.

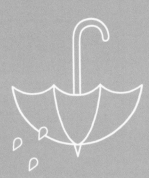

When you walk between different activities during your day — for example, to make a cup of tea or to go to the bathroom — intentionally bring your awareness into feelings in the body as you move: your feet against the floor, your arms swinging by your sides, or the touch of your hand against a door handle.

When you go on a familiar walk, consciously try and notice something new each time that you have not previously heard, seen or experienced.

See if you can build walking into your commute to work or taking your children to school. If it is too far, you could get off the bus or train a stop early or park a little further from your final destination and walk the last bit.

Go for aimless walks, follow your impulses and let yourself be drawn by what catches your interest moment by moment, with no destination in mind. Walk just for the pleasure of walking and the world around you.

If you are feeling adventurous, plan a longer walking trip or hike. There is something pretty special in the simplicity of waking up, taking care of basic needs and walking to a new place. The busy-ness of life may quieten down for a while and allow new perspectives and growth to happen naturally. Plan a walking trip as your next holiday.

When you get the choice, take the stairs rather than the lift. See the extra exercise as a gift to your body rather than unnecessary effort.

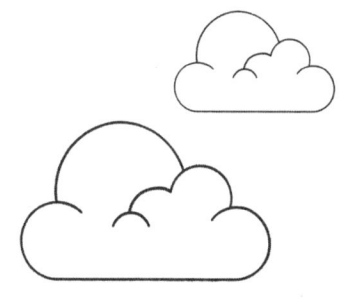

If possible, walk to the shops to get groceries. As well as a way to get outside, this takes us a step back to our ancient roots as hunter-gatherers: rather than taking the car, we are working for our food.

Take a moment at the end of each walk to bring to mind what you have noticed or appreciated during that time.

When you have longer periods of time, plan on going for walks out in the natural world or a park. You could explore some of the practices from this book. You can do this alone or with others, and if you do the latter you may deliberately want to spend some of the time in silence, perhaps even with some space between each person. You can share your experiences of what this is like.

Take pauses when you are out walking to bring your awareness back into the moment. Sometimes you may be forced to stop, such as at a pedestrian crossing. Rather than becoming impatient, use these natural pauses as opportunities for mindfulness.

A WAY TO UNPLUG

Even 20 years ago it may have been hard to imagine how much advances in technology would change our lives. With powerful computers that fit in our pockets, connected to a World Wide Web, we have almost limitless possibilities for information and communication at our fingertips in almost any given moment. This is certainly convenient and brings many benefits, but unchecked it may also have its costs. Technology use can become quite compulsive, even addictive, so we may find ourselves spending more time engaged than we would ideally like, in light of what we most value in our lives and for our own and others' well-being. Without judgement, it can be an interesting inquiry to take time to reflect on our relationship with technology – when and how often we use it, what for, and how it makes us feel. What value does it add to our lives and what costs, if any, does it have? Walking can be a good time to take a break and unplug when trying to cut down or become more conscious of the effect of technology in our lives.

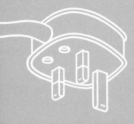

'Our life is frittered
away by detail.
Simplify, simplify.'

HENRY DAVID THOREAU

PRACTICE: SWITCHING OFF

Taking walks can be a time when we can deliberately give ourselves respite and disconnect from the digital world and communications. When you set out for a walk you might like to ask yourself: 'Do I really need to bring my phone? Do I need to be reachable?'

It may also be interesting to notice your reaction to this question. Perhaps it is easy to let go, or maybe there is some resistance. It can be hard to break the habit and any number of reasons may come up for why it is better to take it with you – 'What if so-and-so needs to contact me?' or 'I don't have a watch.' If you notice these thoughts, there is no need to judge them as good or bad, just as bring awareness to what a walk is like if you don't bring a device. Does it affect your experience of the walk? It may be a refreshing break from worry, pressure or distraction.

If you notice strong resistance to unplugging, it may be a helpful reminder that it has only been the past 15 or 20 years that we have had access to such technologies and that the human species generally did okay before this.

STILL PICTURES

Taking pictures with a camera can open us to looking in detail at the world around us, noticing how the light falls perhaps, taking in the landscape, sky and the effect of position and space. Photos provide reminders of what we have seen or experienced and allow us to share some of what we have seen with others. On the flip side, taking photos can further remove us from our experience. Photography can become a means to an end, a way of trying to capture an experience without first living it. I have certainly noticed this tendency in myself at times when I have a camera. When on a walk, do you notice that as soon as you see something of beauty the immediate response is to reach for the camera rather than allow yourself just to appreciate the moment without trying to capture it?

If you like to take a camera with you on walks, the process of taking pictures can become an interesting inquiry. How does having a camera affect your experience of the walk? Does it become impulsive or can the act of taking pictures be done with awareness and mindfulness?

PRACTICE:
MINDFUL PICTURES

If you choose to take a camera out on a walk you might want to make the process of taking photos itself a mindful practice. Here are some ideas that may help.

1. Try and notice the moment in which you decide to take a picture – what is going on in the mind and body: what intention or emotion drew you to this decision.

2. Before you take a picture, first pause and fully take in what you can see. You may even want to turn your body through 360 degrees to take in the entire view.

3. Reflect for a moment on what aspect of the scene you want to capture or draw attention to, or what the mood of the picture might be.

4. When taking the picture, stay in touch with the sensations of your body and your breathing as well as what you are looking at through the lens.

5. When you have taken the picture, pause and take some time to enjoy just looking at the scene in front of you before looking at the picture.

PREPARATION AND SAFETY

Before you embark on your exploration of walking and where it can take you, there are a number of things to bear in mind.

Each reader is unique in many ways and one of these will be your level of experience with walking and being in the outdoors. You may be a seasoned hiker capable of navigation in the mountains and the wilderness or you may find you get lost in your local park. My recommendation is to start from where you are, take care of yourself, stay safe and find the people and resources with which to expand the boundaries gradually of where you can confidently walk without getting lost (for too long!) or coming to any harm. Here are some tips of things to consider when venturing out.

ROUTE

Understanding how to read a map and use a compass allows for good route planning as well as how to avoid getting lost when out on a walk. More recently, GPS and mapping apps offer another way to plan routes and manage navigation.

Be aware that walking speed can vary significantly. An average speed is around 5km (3 miles) per hour. Walking uphill is slower, and by working out elevation gain on a map we can more accurately predict how long a walk will take by adding around one minute for each 10m (33ft) height gain. We can also add on time as we don't typically walk in a straight line – around ten minutes per hour. This does not factor in breaks for food, water or to stop and look at the views. Everyone is different, so it is worth going out and calibrating your own walking speed and times if you want to become more accurate in route planning.

WEATHER

When heading out to more remote or mountainous areas it is important to check a forecast. Weather can change quickly, especially in the mountains, where wind, cloud, rain, temperatures and visibility can fall significantly. It is important to be prepared and take suitable clothing (warm and waterproof) as well as having the tools and knowledge to navigate in reduced visibility. In hot sunny weather it is important to take plenty of water and protect yourself from the sun (hats, sun cream, sunglasses).

Weather conditions and temperature also change as a result of altitude and topography, so if you are going to the mountains, for example, be sure to check a mountain-specific forecast.

COMMUNICATION

Taking with you a means of communicating, such as a mobile phone, can be a good idea in case you get lost or have an accident, even if it is turned off until you need to use it. Letting someone know where you are going, when you plan to be back and what to do if you are not is also worthwhile, particularly if you are going somewhere more remote.

WHAT TO TAKE

This depends on where you plan to walk: the more challenging the terrain and trip length, the more important it is to have the right equipment.

- Supportive boots with good grip
- Clothing suitable for the weather (waterproofs), warm layers, sun hat; remember that wet cotton cools the body down and clings to the skin, so wool or synthetics are preferable)
- Walking poles (especially helpful when carrying a heavy pack)
- First-aid kit (plus whistle)
- Enough water and food
- Suitably sized backpack
- Map and compass (or mapping app on phone with enough battery!)

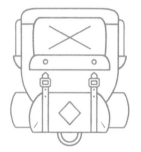

TOWNS AND CITIES

As well as the elements and nature, towns and cities may pose their own risks to take into account, particularly if you are unfamiliar with a place. It might be worth getting local knowledge on where it is safe to walk and at what time of the day or night.

ENOUGH SAID: TIME TO GET OUTSIDE

Walking and spending time out in nature have certainly enriched my life, and I have many memories of special moments while out walking. Of all the places I have walked, from the dramatic and majestic mountains of the Himalayas to the towering old-growth forests of the Pacific North West, the moment which perhaps impacted me the most was walking along a muddy farm track by the side of a lake in Wales. I had walked this path many times and it is not the view or landscape that remains with me but the profound feeling of ease and spaciousness that I experienced. As I walked, for a while it felt like nothing else existed outside of that moment, and my awareness seemed to stretch effortlessly out beyond my usual sense of self, separate from the world out there, and into something more whole, alive and mysterious. This was just an experience and is now a memory, but I feel these moments can shape us and our relationship to life.

I truly hope that at least some of what I have shared in this book will be useful and inspiring for you. If you are already a walker but new to mindfulness, I hope that, like me, finding this new dimension will add richness to your time out walking and stimulate your curiosity.

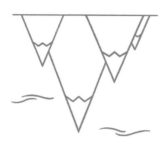

If you already have a mindfulness practice, you might find walking to be a great opportunity to explore and deepen the practice, to take it off the meditation cushion and to integrate it into daily life.

Whatever your background, above all, I hope this book inspires you to get outside and walk, and I wonder what experiences and memories will meet you.

ABOUT THE AUTHOR

I am truly grateful to have been raised by irresponsible parents. Most of my childhood memories are of being outdoors, having the freedom to go out for the day and get lost in the woods or being lovingly dragged up mountains. By age three I had climbed Striding Edge on Helvellyn in winter in wellies and I had been backpacking in Crete and the Austrian Alps before I learnt to read. I am not sure how much I really appreciated it at the time – it was just what we did – but I survived and am now left with a deep lifelong passion for walking and adventure. I discovered the practice of mindfulness in my early twenties and naturally found walking to be a place in which to explore the practice. Mindfulness enriches my experience of walking; I feel more connected, attentive and appreciative of what is going on around me. After working as a researcher and mindfulness teacher at the Centre for Mindfulness Research and Practice at Bangor University for a number of years, I set up Wilderness Minds and dedicated much of my time to my combined passions. Since then, through leading numerous courses and retreats I have had the pleasure of exploring and deepening this practice with countless others. I hope this book captures some of this passion and experience and inspires you to get out there and explore for yourself.

ACKNOWLEDGEMENTS

Thanks to my parents, who, through fearlessly taking me out on adventures from a young age, have instilled a lifelong love for walking and the natural world. Thanks to my mentors and colleagues at the Centre for Mindfulness Research and Practice at Bangor University, who I have learnt so much from and been inspired by, especially Sarah Silverton, Cindy Cooper and Rebecca Crane. Thank you to Heli Gittins and David Elias for supporting me and being a part of Wilderness Minds. To Tamara, for our conversations and support with the writing process, and to Gwladys, my wife, for sharing this life and all your support.

Publishing Director Sarah Lavelle
Editor Harriet Butt
Creative Director Helen Lewis
Designer Emily Lapworth
Illustrator Robbie Porter
Production Controller Nikolaus Ginelli
Production Director Vincent Smith

First published in 2018 by
Quadrille
52–54 Southwark Street
London SE1 1UN
www.quadrille.com

Published in 2018 by Quadrille,
an imprint of Hardie Grant Publishing
www.hardiegrant.com

Text © Sholto Radford 2018
Artwork, design and layout
© Quadrille 2018

Cataloguing in Publication Data:
a catalogue record for this book is available from the British Library.

ISBN: 978 178713 999 9

Printed in China